A Gift, Silently Given

Facing Chronic Illness
With Courage!

Annie Malone Zangari

www.agiftsilentlygiven.com

Book design by www.KarenRoss.com

Note for Librarians: A cataloguing record for this book is available from Library and Archives Canada at www.collectionscanada.ca/amicus/index-e.html
ISBN 1-4251-0518-1

Printed on paper with minimum 30% recycled fibre.
Trafford's print shop runs on "green energy" from solar, wind and other environmentally-friendly power sources.

TRAFFORD PUBLISHING

Offices in Canada, USA, Ireland and UK

Book sales for North America and international:
Trafford Publishing, 6E–2333 Government St.,
Victoria, BC V8T 4P4 CANADA
phone 250 383 6864 (toll-free 1 888 232 4444)
fax 250 383 6804; email to orders@trafford.com
Book sales in Europe:
Trafford Publishing (UK) Limited, 9 Park End Street, 2nd Floor
Oxford, UK OX1 1HH UNITED KINGDOM
phone +44 (0)1865 722 113 (local rate 0845 230 9601)
facsimile +44 (0)1865 722 868; info.uk@trafford.com
Order online at:
trafford.com/06-2276

10 9 8 7 6 5 4 3 2 1

DEDICATION

To my parents,

Marie and Harold Malone,

who modeled the art of joyful hope.

DISCLAIMER

This book is intended to be a comforting, reassuring companion for those who have been diagnosed with a serious chronic illness. It is also intended for family, friends and coworkers who would benefit from a "beginner's book" about living with chronic illness.

Please note that this book is *not* meant, in any way, to be a medical reference book. Therefore, the author and publisher are not responsible for any medical inaccuracies or omissions that may be printed in the text.

Information about any disease included in this book is simply a layman's overview of that illness, and is only meant to describe the outward manifestations that *may occur* with that disease. Any medical issues or questions must be discussed with qualified medical personnel.

IN APPRECIATION

Karen Ross, cover designer, and Kathleen Burgess, editor, for all the extra phone calls, e-mails and general *hand-holding* as this book came together!

PERSONAL THANKS

I would like to acknowledge many people, especially:

My children, for the many months of hearing the words, "I'm working on the book tonight." Special thanks for their reading the chapters and offering suggestions.

Carol Johannes, O.P., for listening to me and guiding me with her wisdom for nearly two decades.

Dr. Stanley Cohan, Dr. Jonathan Pincus, Dr. Peter Wade, and Dr. J. Antonelle (Toni) deMarcaida, for inspiring the chapter, "Does Your Doctor Laugh?"

Anne Zangari for spending so much of her own time formatting and producing the original manuscript, and for being on-call for my many questions.

Linda and Ed McKee for their proofreading, suggestions, and their enthusiasm.

Harold Malone, my brother, for offering honest criticism and helpful suggestions.

Rev. Henry Cody, my Pastor, who shares his gift of joyful hope with *every* person he meets.

All those who shared stories with me as I was writing this book. Their encouragement kept me going.

My husband, Nick, for working countless hours behind the scenes for the duration of this whole project, and who continues to do so!

SPECIAL THANKS

The American Parkinson Disease Association, Inc., which has 65 chapters committed to research and education.

National Parkinson Foundation, Inc., for their dedication to finding the cause and the cure of Parkinson's disease.

Muhammad Ali, who is dedicated to finding a cure, providing treatment, and improving the quality of life for all Parkinson's patients, regardless of financial status, at the Muhammad Ali Parkinson Center in Phoenix, AZ.

Michael J. Fox, for establishing the Michael J. Fox Foundation for Parkinson's Research, the largest nonprofit institution for PD research. Michael has shared so much of his story about young-onset Parkinson's that it is now a household word! (Hopefully, someday to be an *extinct* word!)

A Gift, Silently Given

Facing Chronic Illness With Courage!

Annie Malone Zangari

CONTENTS

INTRODUCTION:

Hold Still! 17

PART ONE: THE INTRUDER

1: The Diagnosis 23

2: Parkinson's disease. 27

3: I'd Seen It Before 30

4: My Turn 34

5: Not Again 39

6: The Choice. 43

PART TWO: THE DAILY EXPERIENCE

7: Getting Up — Just Before Dawn 51

8: Getting Up — Just After Dawn 55

9: Squeak Up!. 59

10: Kitchen Wisdom. 62

11: Does Your Doctor Laugh? 67

12: Oh, My! My Pie! 71

13: If It's Worth Having, It's Worth Asking For . . . 75

14: Bumper Car Blues 77

15: Lost in a Deep Fear 83

16: Sticks and Stones 87
17: Am I Just a Pollyanna? 91
18: Where Do You Get Your P.E.P.? 95
19: About Praise 99
20: The "Secular" and the "Sacred" 103
21: A Chance To Dance 107
22: To Tell Or Not To Tell 110
23: Lace Up Your Sneakers 115
24: Too Old To Dream? 119
25: How About a P.E.P. Group? 123
26: A Simple Prayer 127

CONCLUSION:

27: A New Land 133

ABOUT THE AUTHOR 137

INTRODUCTION

Hold Still!

This book had a stubborn attitude from the first word! It just refused to come together into a unified whole. It was a jumble of emotion, tone and mood. But there's a reason for that.

This is a "beginner's book" (and workbook) about coming to terms with a serious illness that threatens one's life, or *way of life*. It not only speaks to the person who is sick, but also to the spouse, parents, children, friends and co-workers of the person. Many of us are uncomfortable talking about sickness. Hopefully, this book can soften that experience by inserting real people and true stories into the discussion. If you process information through talking (as I do), you may benefit from the questions at the end of each chapter. Add any additional questions that might be helpful to you.

This is a storybook of true tales. Some small details have been changed or combined into one story, and names have been disguised, but these events have been part of my hands-on training over these past several years. These stories have taught me, bit-by-bit, how we can seek comfort in ourselves, with others, and through God.

Let's Talk!

- Have you found yourself in a similar situation with emotions pulling in every direction?

- Have you told any people about your illness?

- Has prayer helped you cope?

PART ONE

The Intruder

CHAPTER ONE

The Diagnosis

A serious medical diagnosis is devastating. The words, "You have __________," are frightening. Did you or someone you love recently get a diagnosis that is really scary? I know what this is like, because I was in that situation myself. Our diseases may be different, but the experiences will have surprising similarities.

Here's what happened to me:

When my four children were very young (9 years; 7 years; 3 years; 16 months), I got up one day and noticed I'd developed a tremor in my hands. I thought it was caused by a medication my doctor had prescribed for an unrelated problem. It turned out there was no connection. Over the next year, three doctors said it was most likely due to stress. I wasn't so sure, but I was willing to believe that it was nothing to worry about.

Months went by. I kept wondering about the tremor. Meanwhile, my symptoms were increasing. They now included: a nearly inaudible voice, clumsy walking, illegible handwriting and relentless fatigue! It was time to get another doctor's opinion.

This doctor said what I'd feared most:"Young-onset Parkinson's disease."

It struck me like a bullet!

Let's Talk!

- What was your diagnosis experience like?

- How did it feel when you were told the diagnosis?

- What could have been done differently to ease the shock of the diagnosis?

NOTES

CHAPTER TWO

Parkinson's Disease

Parkinson's disease (PD) is a degenerative, neurological disorder.

When a person has PD, the brain slowly stops producing dopamine, a neurotransmitter needed for movement. Often a hand tremor is the first observable symptom. Other symptoms may include the following: shuffling walk, poor balance, expressionless face, inaudible voice, weak muscles, "freezing" or the inability to move, and extreme fatigue. Over time, the symptoms increase in number and intensity. Medications eventually are not nearly as effective as they were earlier. PD usually affects people who are 60 or older, but about 5% to10% develop young-onset PD, usually about age 40, or before. There are approximately one million people in the U.S. who have PD.

The medications which are often prescribed for PD are effective for a few hours at a time. PD should be called *The Cinderella Disease.* In that story, the fairy godmother cast a magic spell until midnight. When the spell was broken, Cinderella was left in rags, lying in the road. That resembles life with PD! When the meds are "on," they improve the symptoms; but when the meds wear "off," the symptoms return, sometimes abruptly.

To date, there is no cure.

Let's Talk!

- Are there similarities between living with PD and other diseases?
- Why is there such a feeling of loneliness when an illness is diagnosed?
- Do you feel you would benefit from a support group of people with your illness?

NOTES

CHAPTER THREE

I'd Seen It Before

My Dad, whom we called "Pop," lived with Parkinson's disease (PD) for 13 years. It weighed him down and slowed his steps to the point of "freezing" most of the time.

Pop taught me how to live, and how to die, with an illness. I'd call it a model of *joyful hope*. A person who is full of hope is full of *expectations*. You know - the "glass is half full" kind of person.

Joyful hope acknowledges all truth, but chooses to dwell on positive expectations.

The morning Pop died, I went to see him in hospice before he was moved from his bed. I had just said good night to him hours earlier. He had the same white hospital gown on. But the experience was completely different. Just hours before his death, his hands were limp and he could barely say a word. Sickness seemed to rule the day. But standing there just after he died created a sense of *awe* in me. *I felt no fear*. I could imagine Pop's spirit just got up and left his sick body when his name was called. That room now had the feeling of being sacred. I believed that Pop was finally in the place where his joyful hope could become joyful reality.

At the edge of life and death, thoughts don't follow the same linear patterns that everyday thought follows. As all the memories of being his daughter mingled together, I said, "Pop, thanks for taking me to feed the ducks at Brookville Park when I was little." Why was that memory so vivid?

At that time, I had a new life starting up. I had just married and within a few months, we were expecting our first baby. Our daughter was baptized exactly one year to the day of Pop's death. It was such a different life I was immersed in then. PD was a distant memory. Now was a new chance to weave Pop's joyful hope into my own life.

Let's Talk!

- Have you been with someone at the point of death? What was it like for you?

- Have you found that time is no longer linear when you look back over your relationship with the deceased person?

- Why do we feel awe in the face of death?

NOTES

CHAPTER FOUR

My Turn

My symptoms first started about ten years after Pop died.

As I mentioned, it all began (at least visibly) with a tremor in both of my hands. But there were changes I didn't see.

One friend, who had not seen me in a few years, said she was shocked as she watched me pour a cup of coffee. My movements were slow and deliberate. "You don't realize how much you identify someone by their characteristic way of moving," she later told me.

I had wanted to be an at-home Mom, and those years were wonderful. But I had always intended to return to work when my youngest was school-age. Having recently completed a Master's degree with an emphasis in Business Ethics, I thought it would be exciting to do consulting in that newly-expanding field. It felt especially important because our expenses were increasing as the kids grew. It's so expensive to cover all the constant requests for money from student activities, sports, school, trips, books and other miscellaneous things that come up! In addition, college loomed ahead, not more than four years away.

In the midst of all this, my husband lost his job; he searched for *two years* before finding a new position. This required a relocation, and a significant reduction in corporate responsibilities (and pay!)

As I was putting my resume together about that time, I had to take a realistic look at my health situation. I concluded that on most days: I *planned* to do much; I did much *less* than planned; I was exhausted afterward!

My days were divided into two- or three-hour segments of "on" or "off" energy. The medication was not as reliable any more.The fatigue was not like being tired; *it was like being hit with a stun gun!* Napping during the day, when the kids were having "quiet time," didn't quite make up for the lost sleep at night. (It isn't uncommon to have sleep difficulties with PD.) My head was still thinking I was my old self, but I was beginning to see that I wasn't. Not in some important ways.

What came out of that self-analysis?

I had to admit that my life and my ability to work had been permanently altered.

You know, people say you're never given a burden you are not strong enough to handle. Well, that is not quite the whole story. It doesn't mean that at that time, you are automatically able to handle the burden. I think it's more likely that you are given a chance to have on-the-job training. The new burden is your admission ticket to the "training program," but that's only the beginning. You've got to be willing to work as though your life depends on it, which it may!

I heard someone with PD recently say that the disease robs you of your identity. That is a good description of how it felt at that time – I was too far into PD to feel like my old self, but not far enough into it to realize that the newly emerging version was still very much *me*. Does that make sense?

One of my favorite words of wisdom about living with PD came from my doctor about that time. At the end of an appointment, I asked him how a person could *possibly* lead a normal life with a disease such as this. With a twinkle in his eye, he said simply, "Take a video camera along with you for one day and record what you do. Then watch it. That's your answer."

I guess it's "done in the doing!"

Let's Talk!

- What was your experience like at first?

- Did you have children or other responsibilities that suffered from your being sick?

- What do you think of the video comment?

CHAPTER FIVE

Not Again!

Eight or nine years later, my Mom developed a fast-progressing form of PD, which she had during the last two years of her life. (I understand that this type of PD is very different from the others.) Her recent death has been a painful loss for me, because my Mom had become my PD confidant. On particularly difficult days, I'd call her and say, "Hi, Mom! How's it going?"

Very well, Annie. My legs don't want to move...but it's a perfect day for drying clothes - a nice breeze usually starts up in the late afternoon. Oh, and my garden is beautiful with the flowers in full bloom. I wish we could serve coffee for this little visit!

"That sounds great, Mom. I'll be over in five minutes!"

Mom was well aware that I lived over 100 miles away, and that I wouldn't be coming for coffee, but this child-like humor was enough to get us both laughing. That was the goal! We'd laugh the hardest on the days we were closest to tears. It taught me that those two emotions are not opposites at all. Sometimes, right in the midst of the laughter, I'd choke up a bit: "Mom, this is hard! Do you feel that way, too?"

Yes, Pet, I know. I'm soo sorry!

Let's Talk!

- Do you have a relationship that is unique?

- How difficult is it to feel unconditional love for another person?

- Have you experienced the closeness of the emotions of joy and sorrow simultaneously? Explain, if you can.

-

NOTES

CHAPTER SIX

The Choice

You are given no choice about *becoming* sick or disabled. You only have a choice about how to *respond* to it.

In the beginning, you may feel sorry for yourself, asking, "Why me?" questions. That's a very human response, so don't be impatient with yourself. (Here's where all of those inspirational books you may have read can help!) No matter what age you are, there is a sense of lost possibilities. Whatever you had previously planned is going to change. You feel as though you're missing out - especially when you see someone else doing what you love to do. I feel that way when I realize I can't chaperone a class trip anymore, or travel alone, or swim in the ocean! After spending time (one? two years?) dwelling on those things I couldn't do, I decided to change my approach. I'd been responding to my situation in a reactive manner. It became clear I needed to start thinking more about what I *could* do.

It Was Time to Re-evaluate My Purpose in Life.

There's a desire that is hard-wired into each of us which isn't satisfied until we know where we are going, why we are going there, and what we are planning to do once we arrive. All of us need a role that will make us feel included and *alive*.

God can become our partner in a special way when we are sick, because illness makes a person more humble, and humility seems to be one of God's favorite entryways to our inner self. (Believe me - PD and other debilitating diseases can make you humble in a very short time!) And through God, all things will work together for good. **All things** - including the illness you and I live with - will *work together* for good. I don't understand how this happens, but I believe it. That doesn't mean that a specific request will come true all the time. But there is a kind of peace that I have seen and felt that is beyond our ability to comprehend.

When my daughter was six, she got hit on the head with a golf club. I've never before or since seen a child bleed so much! My neighbor had to call the ambulance because I was in a panic.

When the ambulance arrived, my daughter and I rode in the back. Sirens wailed as we sped to the hospital. She was nearly hysterical and I was petrified. I asked her if she'd like me to say a prayer, and she said she would. I said the words in a conversational manner, telling God that my daughter was hurt, and how very frightened she was. I asked God to stay with her and to *lift her fear*.

When I finished, she stopped crying. She was as calm as if she'd been given a sedative! Amazing!

Later on she said, "Mom, I guess those prayers really do work."

That memory is etched in my heart forever.

In the beginning of my years with PD, my primary purpose was clear-cut: my children were young, and they needed me to be strong. That was, and still is, a powerful motivator. However, now they are growing and they are more independent. I have found an additional purpose: I want to live a life that conveys a sense of humor, hope and joy to anyone feeling crushed by a disease. This book has enabled me to start doing that, and to fulfill a desire to write.

You hear people say, "Attitude is everything." But when you don't feel well, it is hard to know *how* to have a good attitude. I needed more of a blueprint. I tried to break the process into smaller pieces that I could work on each day.

I carry a wrinkled list in my wallet. It says:

Memo to Self

For the rest of my life I want to always:

- Choose hope over fear
- Choose humor over pessimism
- Choose peace over anxiety
- Choose prayer over damning
- NOW…GET WORKING ON IT!

Let's Talk!

- Do you find it difficult to stay positive?

- Do you have a particular purpose that keeps you going?

- What does, "It's done in the doing" mean to you? Is there any part of your life which fits this description?

NOTES

PART TWO

The Daily Experience

NOTES

CHAPTER SEVEN

Getting Up – Just Before Dawn

BZZZZZZZ! SLAM! How can it be time to get up? Maybe you can snoozzzze - NO, you'll be happy you did it - GET UP!

It's still dark, which is the best time. Make that cup of coffee and "take in" the new day.

In the pre-dawn hours, you can watch the morning slowly, gradually evolve from the night. This helps you feel the continuity in your life. (Alarm clocks wake you abruptly and give you the impression that each day is separate—like pieces of peanut brittle in a box.)

Pre-dawn is a time of rituals. A morning ritual or ceremony can be as simple as a moment of silence or a short prayer. It allows you to recognize the sacredness in your life before the day takes hold. *Don't give in to the temptation to empty the dishwasher now. It can wait!* This is a special time to welcome the day. You will feel the difference between a morning that starts with rituals and one that starts with chores. The rituals mark this time as being sacred. And remember, chores will *never* end, so you have to make a choice not to let them steal your best moments.

My morning rituals are simple:

- Open the window in the kitchen. *Listen.* Do I hear birds? They are always the first to know that dawn is coming.
- Pray. In the pre-dawn silence I speak to God in whispers. I feel the need for very few words—Thank you. I'm sorry. Be with us. I love you. God answers in few words, as well—*Be still, and know that I am God* (Psalm 46:10).
- Journal. Simple writing about one or two things which have surfaced in a thought or dream.
- Silence. Notice the *quiet*. Pre-dawn is usually the only time I'll hear it all day.
- Sit quietly, have another cup of coffee, and prepare myself for the day. If I can, 10-15 minutes are wonderful!
- Now, stir all this together, like sugar in my coffee. Then I go and gently wake the children.

Let's Talk!

- Do you have a morning ritual? What is it like?

- Do you have any memories of a particular sunrise or sunset?

- What is your favorite time of day? Why?

NOTES

CHAPTER EIGHT

Getting Up — Just After Dawn

Oh, no! It's 6:45 a.m. I thought I hit "snooze," but I guess I turned my alarm off. Everybody, GET UP! We're LATE! We've got to get out in 20 minutes!

Rushing to the kitchen, I stumble on a sneaker in the doorway. Both the sneaker and I tumble headfirst into Monday morning! "What a mess," I say out loud as I survey the room. I had been so exhausted last night that I had left one pot soaking in sudsy water. That was all it took to create a "starter pile," as my husband calls it. You can clean up a whole room, but if you leave *one* item out of place to finish tomorrow, you have marked the spot where the next mess begins. My starter pile had grown to include cups, cookie crumbs, a sneaker—you know, the one I just tripped on.

The next scene is UGLY! (Parental discretion is advised):

A shrill female voice (mine) is heard, "It's 6: 50; NO—6:50—Get up now! What permission slip? It's due today? A permission slip and a check due on *Monday morning?* Haven't seen your sneakers. Eat SOMETHING! Where did you take your sneakers off? PLEASE get me a pen. What's the dog biting? Forget the Grape Nuts - they take too long to chew. Here's one sneaker under the table. WHAT IS THAT DOG *EATING*? There's a pen on the floor.Your shirt's not ironed. Of course, I'm feeling CRABBY! Forty dollars for a field trip? We're leaving in FOUR MINUTES. He's chewing something pink with laces. We've GOTTA GO, we're five minutes late. He ate your sneaker? GET IN THE CAR. A pen! VROOOOOM! SCREEEECH! VROOOO….

OH, NO! MY GAS TANK IS ALMOST ON "EMPTY"! I used to have mornings like this often. It would stress me out the whole day!

Let's Talk!

- Does this sound at all like your house on occasion?

- When a day starts this way, how does that make you feel?

- Some diseases are much worse when the person is agitated or stressed. This is certainly true of PD. What can you do to prevent this kind of start to the day?

NOTES

CHAPTER NINE

Squeak Up!

Something was stealing my voice. Yours too? At times, my voice was so soft that I felt like a country mouse— all tongue-tied —with nothing but a little "Squeak!" Even in small groups, I had lost the ability to jump in when there was a break in the flow of conversation. (There were times when I had to drink my coffee black because no one heard me ask for milk and sugar!) When I did manage to get a word in, I had grown so used to being mousy that my words were jumbled and unclear. This is a common problem with many illnesses. You begin to lose your voice both physically and figuratively. It's like losing your *Self*.

I knew that I'd have to regain my voice through lots of practice. But that's the hitch—where to get that practice? I found the perfect place. I talk to myself at home when no one is around.

Go ahead—try it. Be foolish! Look the medicine cabinet mirror in the eye and introduce yourself. Have a little chat. Ask yourself questions about your job, your kids, your interests. (Cha, cha, cha....). Now you're talkin'!

Here are a few other points that help with a quiet voice:

- When members of my family find my voice getting too quiet, they let me know it. A reminder such as, "I can't HEAR you" in a teasing manner is helpful.
- Try to speak with inflection in your voice by using high and low tones, especially on the phone. This keeps your voice from becoming a monotone.
- If you are going to participate in a meeting, ask the group leader to periodically ask if anyone has something they want to add. Explain that with your quiet voice, it's hard to jump in when a conversation is fast, loud and opinionated.

With some help, you can become one loud mouse! Come on now—open your mouth, swallow your fears and for heaven's sake, SQUEAK UP!

Let's Talk!

- Have you experienced a *quiet voice*?

- Do people cut you off when you are speaking? If so, what do you do?

- What do you do if you have a very important point to make?

NOTES

CHAPTER TEN

Kitchen Wisdom

I went to a backyard barbeque tonight. Three families were there. Our children are about the same ages, so we have much to share about kids, school and parenting. At one point, the three women in the group went into the house and we had a kitchen chat, shared over the kind of drink that has a little umbrella in it. We'd all had pleasant summers, and we shared many of the details.

Then the conversation turned to me personally. "How's the PD going?" one friend asked.

I answered with one word: "Echhh". This is my way of dismissing the need to talk about it. But wait - why was I doing that when I was with two caring friends? So I took the invitation to talk. Living with PD is like filling the garbage disposal to the brim; talking about it to close friends is like turning the darn thing on!

My voice started to shake and my eyes got teary. I was clueless about what I was going to say, but I knew something was coming out forcefully. "The thing that upsets me the most about PD is worrying about how it impacts my children."

My friend, Carrie, said, "Annie, you have great kids." She said that my kids are growing from this experience by having to take on additional responsibilities around the house or by working part-time jobs to earn money.

My other friend, Lee, said she had seen me with my kids at Starbucks or Dunkin' Donuts getting coffee or a bagel, and she has noticed how much time we spend just being together.

I have had to trade the experiences of chaperoning long class trips, being a full-time room mother, having lots of kids come over after school - all things I used to be able to do - for simpler things. Now I spend most of my time with them taking little trips out to talk about our day, or doing homework at the kitchen table, or watching reruns. These are simple treasures!

I realized I had been blessed by this conversation. We gave each other a three-way hug - all of us with tears in our eyes.

Life's struggles bring us closer. We've all had our own experiences of sickness and of loss. These struggles create a spiritual magnet which draws us toward each other.

Let's Talk!

- Do you find a "kitchen chat" the most comfortable?

- If a parent is handicapped, will children become more independent? How might they grow from the experience?

- What is it that upsets you most about your illness? Do you talk about it?

NOTES

CHAPTER ELEVEN

Does Your Doctor Laugh?

When I was moving out of state a few years ago, I asked my neurologist to recommend a doctor. I was confident in his medical recommendations, but I had another criterion that was important to me. I said I wanted a doctor who laughed! Since my doctor, himself, was the one who made me feel as though I had "PD-lite," he knew exactly what I was asking. He gave me a short list of doctors with notations such as, "Very funny" or "Dry humor" next to the names.

Appointments with some doctors are as impersonal as a walk through a metal detector. The poker-faced doctor will ask a list of disturbing questions about hallucinations, depression, falling, etc., without any trace of empathy.

By contrast, a smiling, laughing doctor makes my semi-annual check-up a booster shot of hope. Even a neurological exam can be humorous. You might find yourself joining in the banter:

"Do you ever hear bells ringing?" - *(No...but please answer that phone!)*

"Are you depressed about having PD?" - *(Am I more sick if I say "yes" or if I say "no"?)*

One cheerful doctor started every appointment by asking me to list everything that was going well with my health. Only after hearing the positive list would he ask for any problems I might be having. Psychologically, this was ingenious! I still make a list of what is going well and I read it to my doctor at the beginning of each appointment. It helps me feel optimistic about things I may never have noticed. For example, maybe I have been sleeping more soundly, or perhaps my walking may feel stronger. My doctor comments on how good it is to hear these things, and he notes them in my file. Otherwise, the only comments that get entered into the file are negative ones.

The bottom line is: if your doctor makes you feel like a *sick person*, perhaps you should find a new doctor. Although it's unspoken, this is the worst diagnosis you can receive. It is the one which will stick in your head. Rather than feeling like a person with a full life, who happens to have a chronic disease, you will feel like a *walking disease.* Period.

I have had both kinds of doctors and I know the difference. You *deserve* a doctor who laughs.

Let's Talk!

- Does your doctor laugh?

- What personal qualities put you at ease with a doctor?

- Have you had a doctor who made you feel like *nothing*?

NOTES

CHAPTER TWELVE

Oh, My! My Pie!

Let's face it. I don't eat many meals balanced on my lap anymore. In case you haven't tried it in a while, you may be surprised at how tricky this can be with PD or some other "shaky" disease.

A friend is hosting a buffet dinner. It's a comfortable setting with people who make me feel relaxed. However, there are challenges ahead.

The meal is being served on good china and with long-stemmed wine glasses. (*Easy, girl! You know what to do.*) I could skip the wine (*No way*) or ask for help carrying it (*Why not?*). I hold the plate in my left hand and serve myself all the one-handed foods (such as rolls, mashed potatoes, chicken tenders, olives.) Okay—I'm set up in a sturdy chair with a small table in front of me. My "junior" foods require no cutting. There's a conversation going on next to me. I'm going to try to talk *and* to keep eating at the same time. I can almost remember how to do this.

After dinner, my host brings me a piece of pie and a cup of coffee. No problem. The concept is the same. Move the pie to the left hand and balance it there briefly. Put the sugar in the coffee and stir. Pick up the fork. (My right hand is showing off—not even a tremor.) Now for the pie.

Doing great, right? *Wrong!* Before my right hand can get to it, my left hand turns my pie plate sideways, and the pie vanishes. There lies my key lime pie, on the rug! I don't know what to say. *I feel like I've just been cut from the team.*

I've done my "pie trick" at a few get-togethers. Some social situations will always be hard, but here's some advice: If you are in need of special assistance—and if you're dropping pie, you are—it's up to *you* to let the host know what would help. It is hard to be outspoken because no one wants to be a bother. However, being shy about your physical needs is no longer an option.

Remember - *You (the person with the illness,) are the expert, and you will set the tone for everyone else.*

P.S. For those who have asked me how to offer help, I'd say only this: BE SPECIFIC.

- *Don't say:* "If there's anything I can do let me know…" or "Give me a call if you need groceries…"
- *Do say*: "I'd like to bring bagels for your kids this Thursday morning" or "I'm going to ________

Store about 10:00 this morning, and I can easily get you a bag of groceries. I'll call you in twenty minutes for your list. OK?"

Now, would you like another piece of pie?

Let's Talk!

- Does your illness cause you to stay home more often than you would like?

- Would you find it easier to ask for help if you were going to the home of a person who is also handicapped in some way?

- Can you think of any embarrassing, funny or surprising event that happened to you in a group?

CHAPTER THIRTEEN

If It's Worth Having, It's Worth Asking For

I remember my Mom and I would pull up in front of Jess White Cleaners every Monday when I was almost six years old. We would drop off a few long-sleeved white shirts to be laundered, saying, "Light starch; Wednesday, please." Each time the smiling clerk would pull out a lollipop basket and offer me one. I'd shyly take a red one and say "Thank you" to the lady. It's one of my fondest memories.

Fast-forward two years. I was eight years old and I still loved lollipops (purple ones by then.) One week Mom added a new twist to our Jess White Cleaners routine. I was horrified when I heard the new terms! Mom would stay in the car, not more than ten feet from the counter, and I had to bring in the shirts and say, "Light starch; Wednesday, please," *all by myself!* I protested vehemently, but when Mom decided it was time to take the next step in learning life skills, it was useless to try and change her mind.

Slowly, I dragged my reluctant self into the cleaners. Then the most awful thing happened—at least to my way of looking at it. I dropped the shirts on the counter, gave the instructions, and waited for my lollipop. But the woman said nothing. I waited a few seconds longer, the way my dog waits when he's done a new trick. But the woman said nothing. NOTHING. So I left.

When I got back in the car and told my Mom, she said to go back and politely ask the lady if I might have a lollipop. I'd rather have been dipped in light starch than do that. Mom simply said, "If it's worth having, it's worth asking for."

Thus began many years of hearing that dreaded sentence in countless situations:

- telling a teacher I thought there was a mistake on my test grade
- asking shopkeepers if they would purchase an ad in our school yearbook
- inviting a new friend to our house for the first time

I could hear Mom's answer even before I'd tell her my latest quandary: "If it's worth having, it's worth asking for."

The value of that maxim didn't end in childhood. In fact, I'm reminded of it frequently now that I have to ask for help with tasks I used to do myself. Recently,

I needed someone's help to solve a problem. Mom was sick and I couldn't drive the three hours to visit her anymore. My family couldn't get there as often as I liked. For a few months, I mulled over the problem and finally decided to take action.

Maybe someone at my parish rectory might know of a parishioner who made that trip routinely. Yes! I was given the name of a woman, Sally, who did. When I called her and explained where I needed to go, it turned out Sally was from the same hometown, and she had been a classmate of my brother. (She asked me if I had been the little sister who used to tag along. *That's me!*)

As with so many problems which seem like a roadblock, if you ask for help, the new solution is better than the old one. Not only did I find a driver, but I have a new friend who has known my family for many years.

When my Mom died recently, I was grateful to Sally for writing a touching note about what a beautiful, gentle woman Mom was. Sally wrote about how pleased she was to have seen and talked to Mom just before her death.

Feeling deeply grateful for the important role Sally played in the last few months of Mom's life, I'm reminded once again:

"If it's worth having, it's worth asking for...."

That sentence is like denim—it goes with everything!

Let's Talk!

- Were you encouraged to speak up as a child?

- Do you encourage your children, grandchildren, etc., to be politely outspoken?

- When do you find it difficult to ask for what you need?

CHAPTER FOURTEEN

Bumper Car Blues

Aren't bumper cars great? One of the best summer pleasures is to be at an amusement park near dusk (when lines are shortest) and to go on the bumper cars several times without waiting. When drivers race toward my car, I still get a rush. The real joy is in being able to break all the rules you have to follow in real life!

I love to cause "accidents" when I'm in a bumper car. First, I choose a slow-moving target up ahead, I look for a clearing, and then I gun it. A direct hit and a surprised look on the face of the other driver always makes me laugh. Invariably, another driver will sideswipe me seconds later, and often another crash will turn my car hopelessly around. Then comes the real challenge of getting back on track, and in the spirit of it all, doing it once again.

However, the last time I went, my sides actually *hurt* after getting knocked around a few times. I had not noticed *pain* other years. After a multiple vehicle accident, my car was immovable. The other cars got rolling, but I was still spinning my wheels. I wasn't enjoying the challenge. What had happened to the laughter?

Could the problem be PD? There was no good reason PD would affect my bumper car driving. But this kind of thinking *resembles* logic just enough to get you and me in trouble.

It says:

> *If PD (or another disease) sometimes affects my performance, and if I am not performing something well, then PD must be responsible.*

Beware! This is faulty logic. Your illness may have nothing to do with your performance. You might just be having an off day. Even the best athletes have days when they're not at their best.

Find out if other people with PD (or your disease) have trouble with a particular activity.

Want a few suggestions?

- A good rule is to give up *nothing* until you are absolutely sure your medical problem is not compatible with it.
- Ask a trusted friend if he or she thinks your health is preventing you from "going for it."
- Try the activity again soon. See if you have the same problem. Bet you don't!

You know what? I still love bumper cars!

PD? What's that got to do with it?

Let's Talk!

- What activity is like "bumper cars" for you?

- Have you given up some activities you knew were not safe to continue? How has that affected you?

- When you find a special activity has become too strenuous, do you try and think of an alternative? Can you think of an example?

NOTES

CHAPTER FIFTEEN

Lost in a Deep Fear

August 30, 2000 (journal entry):

I hit a real low point yesterday in the afternoon. I was feeling very low energy and overwhelmed with everything.... Nick and I prayed together. I cried...Maybe God is leading us out of this dark valley, ...but it doesn't feel that way. We (feel) forgotten. Abandoned. I can't take any more.

How much more, Lord?

Some days PD scared me, and the feeling might linger for days. No silver linings. No respite. At times I was lost in a deep fear.

You don't have to have an illness to know what it's like to be "lost in a deep fear." At such a time, keeping up the dialogue with God may seem useless. It's as though He has left you alone in the woods. At those times, I try *bombarding* God with prayer, asking over and over for the joy of feeling His presence. Remember, there is no such thing as being a "pest" in

God's eyes. If we were to wheedle a human this way, we'd be told to back off! But God doesn't work that way. Every word we utter, pleading to feel God's presence, is breaking down the wall we are facing. God wants us to break through even more than we want to! Picture being a parent whose two-year-old is locked in the car. How frantic would you feel? God is like that with us.

One incident stands out for me. I had been depressed for several days, and I desperately needed to feel connected with God. It was New Year's Day. Taking a long walk, I talked silently to God, asking over and over to let me experience the deep peace only He can offer. This was no finely-worded prayer! I must have sounded like a whining child. Repeatedly, I reminded God that I felt unable to continue without that peace. It seemed I did all the talking - and I went on for a long time!

Just as I was coming back to my own street, two doors away from home, I had a sensation of something inside me being broken open. The closest image I can use to describe it is the way a large tree branch might crack in a storm. At the time I didn't know whether this was anything significant or not. It turned out it definitely was. My fear, isolation and despair were lifted. What a happy day that was!

(There are many times prayers are not answered in that powerful way. Remember, I'd been praying for days for a respite, and none seemed to be there. God's timetable is so different from ours!)

Let's Talk!

- Have you had the experience of being "lost in a deep fear?"

- Was it related to having an illness or another trauma?

- Why do you think God seems so distant at times?

NOTES

CHAPTER SIXTEEN

Sticks and Stones

My kids have been taught to never, ever make fun of someone with any kind of handicap. But somewhere along the line, my family decided that it was *open season* on teasing me about PD. This has been a release for me and for them, because it gives us the gift of laughter.

The funniest jokes have come in relation to my "Parkie Shuffle," as the kids call my walking. My son will say, "This is Mom's *Speedy* Parkie shuffle," and he'll slide his feet along the floor in a locomotion kind of step, but he remains in the same spot. He'll try harder, moving his arms and his legs, but he's going nowhere! I always burst out laughing, "You look so FUNNY!"

My most recent PD problem involves not being able to turn myself around when I am in a tight corner. It requires pivoting on one foot, and circling with the other. When the kids imitate this movement, it looks like the first foot is nailed to the floor.

A short while ago, I was explaining this teasing to my friend and her daughter, who is a young mother. I could tell her daughter was surprised that I am comfortable with this. Years ago, I would have considered it "making fun," and I probably would not have approved either. My friend, however, laughed as I told the story. Maybe, as we get older, the beauty of laughter becomes increasingly clear to us.

So go ahead—have a good laugh at yourself. Have a few embarrassing moments and stories you can comfortably share when someone asks how you are, and you don't want to be too serious. Humor shrinks the problem to a manageable size.

If you're comfortable with it, ask your kids or a friend to do a funny imitation of the way you do something, such as putting on your shoes, or calling the family to supper, or—one of our favorites—"Here's Mom trying to get out of the recliner."

Your family may have trouble talking about your illness, but this lets them express their feelings through humor. Seeing you laugh lets them know it's OK to laugh, too. As you find more humor in your life, your burdens will lighten up, just a bit at a time.

Illness is no joke, but it certainly can be funny!

Let's Talk!

- Do you find it difficult to laugh about your health problems?

- What lightens your burdens when you are low?

- Do you believe in the power of prayer?

NOTES

CHAPTER SEVENTEEN

Am I Just a Pollyanna?

Someone asked me if all my emphasis on laughter and humor could be viewed as a "Pollyanna" philosophy—that all you have to do is make a joke and the problem will go away. No! That simplistic view will not carry anyone very far in dealing with an illness.

Medicine is now discovering that when the *whole person* is treated, no matter what the disease, the outcome is far beyond what was thought possible even ten years ago. These are the areas I have tried to strengthen:

- Exercise
- Personal relationships (family and friends)
- Prayer
- Writing
- Laughter/Humor

Humor is just one ingredient. It is important because *it allows family and friends to become part of your struggle. Humor allows people to know they don't have to tiptoe around your health problem.*

I didn't come to this realization myself. My husband pointed out to me that while the patient is the only one who "needs treatment," the entire family lives with the disease.

The children, spouse, other relatives and friends of the person have questions and fears, but they frequently don't express them. They feel they have to take their cues from the patient, who may be totally self-absorbed. That is where humor comes in. It provides a door through which others can enter the world of the patient, and even briefly control the situation by creating laughter. Children can join in the laughter and joking. Anything that makes the children feel like a part of the inner circle creates security for them.

Humor is just plain good for everyone!

Let's Talk!

- Do you know someone who is able to combine humor and illness?

- Can humor be perceived as insensitivity?

- Humor does not have to be specifically about the disease. How about taking the family to a funny movie just to lighten the mood?

NOTES

CHAPTER EIGHTEEN

Where Do You Get Your P.E.P.?

Do not face your illness alone. We all need at least one person who is always there for us, even if that person lives a thousand miles away.

This person cares deeply about what you are going through and offers consolation *you can count on*. You don't have to *prove* that you deserve it. We are created as social beings, and sickness is meant to be shared.

I have found three indispensable qualities in a friend when it comes to truly helping you cope with illness:

Patience in listening to your story—someone who lets you talk about it as long as you need to talk.

Empathy in understanding how you feel—someone who "empathizes" tries to actually feel what you are feeling. The last thing you need at this time is a friend who judges your feelings or who condemns you for your mistakes.

Praise—someone who offers praise about how you are coping with the illness. This quality may surprise you, but it has strong healing power! A chronic disease is all day, every day. You get very little feedback about how you are doing, except for a doctor's visit. A friend who will say, for example, "I admire you because you show a lot of courage," actually conveys courage to you when you might be feeling anything but courageous! Patience. Empathy. Praise. These are qualities you will need in at least one friend, whom we will call your P.E.P.

Where do you find a P.E.P.?

You may be lucky enough to have discovered one in a relative or friend, or a neighbor who talks to you over the fence. If you have one who lives far away, well, then *pick up that phone.* Tell the person how precious his or her encouragement is to you. Don't be afraid of sounding silly. You can trust this relationship. It also can be a reciprocal friendship. Maybe *you* can be *their* P.E.P., too.

Let's Talk!

- Do you have a P.E.P.?

- Can you describe your relationship with this person?

- Which is the most difficult trait for you to show—patience, empathy or praise?

NOTES

CHAPTER NINETEEN

About Praise

A few close friends said they were surprised to see "Praise" included among the top three qualities of a P.E.P. (Patience, Empathy and Praise). They said it was a good thing to learn, because the person on the outside doesn't know how praise will be received. They hesitate, too, because praise can sound insincere.

Keep in mind that the person with a chronic illness lives with that handicap constantly. It is a lonely drama which has no script and no audience. That means no feedback. Observers may feel they are not in a position to comment since they don't have the disease themselves. But think of all the things about which you can comment. Just observe:

Maybe you see your friend struggling to cut her food in a restaurant. It takes "guts" to even go out in public when you have such a handicap. Don't hesitate to say you admire her courage and the fact that she doesn't let anything stop her. *Be willing to make a gift of praise.* It may be the only emotional food that keeps her going that day! Without your input, she might have decided this was the last time she is going to go out for lunch because it's too embarrassing and too exhausting. Throw her a line!

Write a note to a handicapped friend. Tell her what you admire in her struggle. Be specific. Tell her what you've observed and why you admire that quality. Remember, your note will probably be taped to the refrigerator later on - so make it encouraging!

Don't hesitate if you feel your friend is a private person who would not want much ado made about him. My father was the most humble person I have ever known. Yet, when he died, we found a little notebook in his dresser where he kept brief thoughts and comments. One touching entry said the nun in charge of Outreach in his church during his illness said he was a "parish treasure." He got so much joy from that simple comment!

Praise. It costs nothing, but it's priceless!

Let's Talk!

- Are you comfortable when you receive praise?

- Do you praise other people?

- Why is praise stressed so much more today than it was years ago?

NOTES

CHAPTER TWENTY

The "Secular" and the "Sacred"

My outlook on life has become increasingly spiritual, and here's the reason why.

My diagnosis was an awful blow to me. This intruder had crept in during the night and had stolen my future. (That's what it felt like!) It was unbelievable. Not only that, but I felt so alone. Not even my doctor knew what it was really like. Many times, I didn't know how I was going to make it through the day.

My faith didn't seem strong enough to carry me, but I knew this was my only chance of finding meaning in my new situation. It was at that time I wrote in my journal:

Nov. 21, 1995

"I have become aware of how fragile life is and how quiet faith is.

I want God to speak louder."

It became important to find the sacred meaning in the secular events of my life. If I could find purpose in all aspects of life, then I could make sense of losing what had been lost - the freedom to choose my own future.

It still is a struggle some days. There are times I feel envious of others. And, other days I wonder what things would have been like, if only...

And then there are days I see sacred beauty in my life, beauty that I know I would not have previously noticed. Now, I'm talking about really tiny events - for example, I now have time in the morning to cook old-fashioned oats, and I can actually stick around to "stir occasionally," as the instructions recommend. I spent the first 40 years of my life always rushing, running late, and eating instant oatmeal. (Instant oatmeal will never be "sacred" for me - I'm sorry!!)

During the years that Pop was sick, whenever things got too tough, both my parents would get in the car and go out for a hot fudge sundae. Just even hearing the words "hot fudge sundae" put them in a joyful frame of mind. They'd go to their local ice cream parlor, see people they knew, chat a bit, eat their ice cream - and then they'd be ready to take on their next hurdle. When I'd go along with them, I could tell that a transformation had taken place. I don't know that I would have used these words then, but I would now say that the little trip out for ice cream had converted the situation from a burden to a simple blessing - from the secular to the sacred. They were masters at doing that!

Another aspect of this secular/sacred melding: I've found that God has a sense of humor. (At least I think there are two of us laughing!) There are many Sundays I have trouble walking in the communion line with "The Twins"(i.e., my troublesome feet) - they are like stubborn, adolescent kids who decide when and if they are going to walk. One week, when they had been especially troublesome, I went to the book of prayer requests in our church and simply wrote: "The Twins." I knew no human reading the book would have a clue as to who these twins were, but I was pretty sure God was amused. Just picturing it lightened my frustration and embarrassment. Now, I often write that same petition in the book, and no one else has any idea who they are! I imagine the Pastor must see them in the book week after week, and think: those darn twins are at it again!

Here's one last thought on this topic of the secular morphing into the sacred -

A few years ago, I was on the mailing list for a monastery that made the best butter crunch candy I've ever eaten. Waiting for the candy to arrive was really torture for me, but always worth the wait! It felt like a "sacred" experience - I'd eat the candy while I read the enclosed brochure describing monastic life! Those nuns all looked so joyful and peaceful (and *thin*) as they made that candy. Each year, after I had eaten almost the entire box, my experience became definitely "secular," as I faced the stomachache and the extra pounds! At that point, I guess I was on my own!

Let's Talk!

- Do you look for the "sacred" in the "secular" parts of life?

- When do you find it most difficult to do that? (e.g., when things are going well, or when they are going badly?) Why does God allow us to have to endure hardships in life?

- Do you believe suffering can offer an opportunity for deeper joy?

CHAPTER TWENTY ONE

A Chance To Dance

I love to dance! Nothing fancy. Just having a chance to listen to music and to move my feet is wonderful therapy for my body - and my outlook.

For three years, I've taken the "The Twins" (my feet) to Line Dance classes in our community center. "We" have taken the class six or seven semesters.

Dancing has brought some special people into my life. My buddy in class is a little lady, Tina, who is in her 80's. She is as peppy as a Super Ball. Tina takes dance classes so she can remain limber for her two bowling leagues, one of which she has been in for 40 years! Our instructor, Callie, has given me a role model for how dancing should look and *feel*. She stresses the importance of smiling and graceful body movements, which is great for me, because my footwork is not so good!

Sorry to say, my dancing has been problematic lately, and I wonder if I can continue much longer. I've had trouble with *freezing*, an inability to move my feet some days. It is a new PD symptom for me and one which makes it difficult to dance.

Recently, Callie played my favorite waltz, one I usually sing along with quietly. It's a four-wall dance, so every eight bars of music, the dancers rotate one-quarter turn. Since I was on the outside row, every time the class rotated in my direction, I was in full view of everyone.

When the music began, I kept time with my hands, as we do in class. Suddenly, it happened. My feet refused to move. They wouldn't even walk *off* the dance floor! I thought everyone must be looking. Even after all this time, I feel embarrassed whenever a new symptom starts. Pride dies hard! I couldn't wait for class to end. I left quickly when it finally did end.

The next week I didn't go back. Weighing the pros and cons of continuing was upsetting. My pride insisted that the class would be intolerable if my feet froze again. On the other hand, maybe the joy of swaying to the music would be enough. *Who says I can't take a dance class just because my feet don't move some days?* Finally, it seemed I should give it one more chance.

The day I went back, Callie played my favorite waltz again. This time "The Twins" were, inexplicably, on best behavior, and they danced effortlessly. I said a prayer of thanks for the joy of it all as I wiped my eyes with my hand.

Since that day when I couldn't dance, I've had a deep appreciation of all the days I can dance.

Yes, this is a crossroads, but I think the only answer is to keep on dancing. It gives me a chance to feel graceful some of the time, and that makes it worthwhile.

As if she were reading my mind, Tina said to me recently, "When I'm at home, I can think of so many reasons not to come. I have to *push* myself to get out and to keep on going."

"Yes, Tina, me too!"

So let's just put on our dancing shoes.

Let's Talk!

- Is there some special part of your life you have had to give up due to your illness?

- Do you avoid some things you enjoy for fear of looking awkward?

- Why is it so hard to let go of pride?

CHAPTER TWENTY TWO

To Tell Or Not To Tell

I have told people I have PD ever since the day I found out.

It seemed the most comfortable thing to do. There was no reason to hide my diagnosis. Talking helped me to process it and made me feel less alone. Plus, it did my confidence good to have someone say, in response to hearing that I have PD, "Really? I couldn't tell *at all*."

Now, years have passed. For those who don't know exactly why I'm shuffling and clumsy, I will mention it casually, sometimes saying I have the "Cinderella Disease," that is, when my meds wear off, the spell is broken. I try to schedule my appointments for "on" times. However, this is not at all foolproof. Last week I was attending an evening function at my son's school. It ran from 7:00 P.M. to 9:00 P.M. About 8:30, I could feel my feet get heavier. That meant I had to leave, even though the spell should have lasted longer!

I guess it's a question of timing. When you decide to tell people, do you want the response to be, "I had no idea," or would you rather wait and have the response—which would probably remain unspoken—be something like, "I *wondered* what was the matter with you!"

This reminds me of the woman who started lying about her age. She told people she was ten years older than she actually was. That way, people always commented, "You look so young!"

So would you rather be told you look terrific for someone with PD (or some other illness) or have people wonder why you look so wobbly for a person with nothing the matter?

Let's Talk!

- Have you had other situations in your life in which you felt torn about admitting a problem? How did you resolve the situation(s)?

- Do you find you don't want others to see you when your meds are not at their best?

- Are people (cashiers, drivers, people in lines) sometimes impatient with you?

NOTES

CHAPTER TWENTY THREE

Lace Up Your Sneakers

Once a year, there's a PD walk-a-thon in which my family and I take part. Early on a Sunday morning, we all head out for the event, which is held in a local mall. From the moment we drive up, I feel the charge of energy and goodwill. People wearing "Parkinson's disease" T-shirts greet us, and there's a smile and a good word from every person. Our kids love the free snacks and bottled water. The Starbucks coffee is another free treat I gratefully accept. After a few minutes, we begin walking.

The walk-a-thon consists of as many laps as you can do around the mall. There are people with walkers, speedy young kids, grandparents with teens, and every level of walking ability.

As we walk along, counting laps, my husband and I always get into a conversation that sums up the year in terms of how we, as a family, have dealt with PD.

Each day every one of the people present at the walk-a-thon lives with PD, just as we do. Most days there is not one other person whom we'll see who has the disease. *PD is a solo event.* Even a support group only meets sporadically. However, this is not the case on walk-a-thon day. People with PD predominate. I am proud to be part of the group because they just keep going!

I am sure caregivers find consolation in seeing other caregivers. Children are relieved to see there are other kids whose parent or grandparent has PD, too.

I look around and see lots of folks who are struggling with more advanced states of PD than mine, and it gives me courage. If they can persevere, then so must I. When individuals speak at the brief meeting following the walk, I am impressed with how knowledgeable they are. These leaders blend practicality with large doses of hope—a dynamic combination!

The sense of unity created by the walk-a-thon works its magic in all of us. It reminds us we are all part of an extended family. There's new energy in abundance, which will see us through our dark days.

See you next year!

Let's Talk!

- Have you been able to attend an event like a walk-a-thon?

- How did it make you feel?

- Did you feel energized into action? In what way?

NOTES

CHAPTER TWENTY FOUR

Too Old To Dream?

My daughter and I were returning from a video store. She needed to pick up a DVD to prepare for a role in a play. As we were driving home, she said, "The big difference between you and me is I can still dream and you can't."

"Why can't I dream?" I asked, wondering what I was missing.

"I can dream about possibilities," she said. "Will I be a millionaire? Will I have kids? Will I become an actress?"

"You're too old to dream dreams like that," she added.

That conversation got me thinking. A decade ago, when the doctor confirmed my diagnosis with the words, "Parkinson's disease," all I could see were limitations stretching out before me. As ten years have gone by, I've had to let go of some dreams: teaching school again; returning to graduate school; going into the field of business ethics.

Not that there is no way to get started in those endeavors, but rather it has become a question of choosing my *highest* priorities. Since PD limits my energy, it limits my choices. That means only my most precious dreams can be pursued. At first, this felt like an awful limitation. Now I see that limitations give me the freedom to let go of "second-string" dreams.

While I was mourning the old dreams which were dying, new dreams were being born. I've wanted to write a book for years, but I lacked the confidence that I had something to say. I don't lack confidence anymore. Why? The very thing that has forced me to forfeit some dreams has offered me new ones that I couldn't have imagined. Writing about my experience with PD has given my life a new purpose. I'm hoping it will resonate with others who have let go of some of their fondest dreams, too.

Dreams present possibilities for new growth. This statement reminds me of an article I read that said some of the wildfires out west get so hot that seeds, which have been dormant for over 100 years, are cracked open and they sprout! Just imagine a parallel scenario in your life. Is it possible that seeds which have been dormant for decades are being cracked open by the "heat" of your illness? Look around. What beckons to you?

The next time I get a chance to talk with my daughter about dreams, I'm going to tell her mine are alive and well and giving me hope. Maybe she will even want to hear some of them.

Let's Talk!

- What seeds have been dormant in you for years?

- Will your health issues help or hinder those seeds from sprouting?

- What important part of your life have you had to give up, if any?

CHAPTER TWENTY FIVE

How About a P.E.P. Group?

Not everyone wants to share their personal details about having an illness, but for some, this is the way they can process their experience. A small group can be wonderful for people who want to share, in a social and spiritual context, their experience of being ill or having a chronic disease.

As you know, chronic illness cuts a person off. When I was diagnosed with PD, I didn't know *one person* who had a young family and a chronic disease. My doctor didn't know anyone I could talk to, either.

Eventually, I met a friend who had children the same ages as my own, who had some health issues of her own. Another friend joined us and we formed a small group (Pray and Play), which lasted for about three years.

This is all it takes to start a group:

- Materials. This book can be used for a group. The chapters are short, there are discussion questions at the end of each chapter, and the material deals with chronic illness. We used to laugh and say if the chapter couldn't be read during the traffic lights on the way over to the meeting, then it was too long.
- Find one, two or three interested people. Ask around. If you are fortunate enough to know others with your illness, that is terrific; but it is not necessary. Try putting an announcement in the Sunday bulletin at your church to see if there is interest in a group.
- After the first meeting, people will know if the group has "chemistry." Then you can decide to meet again or to have it be a one-time get-together.
- Either take turns at the members' homes, or meet at the same home each time. A coffee shop is great, too.
- Remember that P.E.P. stands for Patience, Empathy and Praise, as you share experiences together.
- Open and close with a non-denominational prayer if members are of different faiths, or a conversational prayer if there are members who feel comfortable doing this.
- Here is one last bit of advice - like a secret ingredient in your mother's oatmeal cookies: Just before the group arrived at my home, I'd say a prayer asking

the Spirit to be present with us and to be felt by each of us. I'm convinced there was always a serenity during those get-togethers which no one could put a finger on!

Let's Talk!

- Would you like to be part of a P.E.P. Group?

- Do you find most people experience similar emotions even though their disease can be very different from your own?

- One of the ways God communicates with us is through other people. Does your P.E.P Group seem conducive to this movement of the Spirit?

CHAPTER TWENTY SIX

A Simple Prayer

Dear Friend,

This is difficult. It is a burden waiting to be picked up and carried every day of my life. Exercise, nutrition, vitamins, affirming self-talk and a positive outlook can lighten the burden, *but this disease doesn't go away*. There are some dark days when this realization feels like too much to handle. On those days, I can't face my reality. So what do I do then? I lock my bedroom door. I sit in a comfortable chair. I put my head in my hands, and I let the tears come. I cry my eyes out. (That really seems to help.) And then I pray a simple prayer: "Lord, it's Annie. I need you. Don't leave me."

God wants to help us with our sorrow. All we have to do is ask. At those times, I let my deepest concerns and my tiniest inconveniences—the whole package—be expressed. I might say, "Lord, my walking is getting slower, and I almost fell yesterday; my meds haven't been working so well; I didn't get more than five hours of sleep last night; my kids need me to be a healthy mother to keep up with their busy lives; I'm weary and I can't see Your face in all of this. Are You there?"

I find this type of conversational prayer especially helpful. As I express my concerns, desires, etc. to God, I am listening to myself, and am often hearing the problem for the first time. Think about it. Have you ever been upset or angry about something, but you didn't know *what?* Maybe you're about to cry, but you haven't got a clue *why*?

That's the time for a conversation with God. Just start talking - when you're alone - and tell God you don't know what's the matter. Keep talking! Chances are it will become clearer as you speak. Prayer acts like a garden tool that loosens the soil so a plant can grow with plenty of room.

To finish what I was saying about prayer, when I've finished, then I wait. And I wait. And I wait a little longer. Most often, nothing happens right away. But something always happens. Possibly an article in the paper will cheer me up. Maybe someone will just happen to call. Or one of the kids will get me laughing. Answers come in simple ways.

This process of conversing with God is very powerful. It has carried me this far, and it will carry me home, some day, I am sure.

Let's Talk!

- What do you do when your health issues become too heavy for you to carry alone?

- Do you hesitate to tell God about your negative feelings—anger, feeling forgotten, despair about whether you'll be able to handle your illness?

- Does it seem that God often answers prayer in a different way than you'd expected? Explain.

NOTES

Conclusion

NOTES

CHAPTER TWENTY SEVEN

A New Land

For many years, I've kept a personal journal which contains just about anything I think, dream, or pray about. In writing this book, I've re-read old journals from the period of time my symptoms first began. Something unusual recently surfaced. It was a journal entry written *eight weeks before any symptoms of PD started*!

It's a prayer meditation:

September 12, 1995:

He is leading me off the boat we've been on during a terrible storm. We are in a new land. I'm carrying baggage. He's walking with me. I'm weary, but He is...encouraging. We are going to a new place. I am tired and afraid. I don't want to go. He is gentle, never rushing me. Where?...

I think God gave me an inkling that something frightening was coming, but also the reassurance that I was in good hands. I never went back to that journal entry until all these years later.

You know what else strikes me? Here I am, more than ten years later, going through a stack of journals, and the date on one entry tells me that God had given me a powerful gift which I didn't recognize all those years ago. It was so understated - either I'd see it, or not.

The fact that I didn't recognize its significance back then doesn't change it - I just didn't have the eyes to see it. But now I can observe this short entry and recognize that this is probably one of thousands of little messages along the way that were tiny glimmers of the sacred meaning of my life.

How typical of God to work in that way: a gift, silently given, not even acknowledged until many years later. And signed only,

"Guess Who?"

Let's Talk!

- Have you experienced a time when God seemed to be working silently in your life?

- Do you look for little signs of God's presence in your day?

- Have you ever experienced a premonition during prayer?

NOTES

ABOUT THE AUTHOR

Annie Malone Zangari is a hands-on expert when it comes to living with chronic disease. Annie, herself, developed young-onset Parkinson's disease after the birth of her fourth child, when all of her children were under the age of ten. Her father and mother both had Parkinson's disease. Through years of observing her parents, Annie learned how they converted their daily struggle into a life of hope. Their modeling became the basis of *A Gift, Silently Given*.

Annie holds an undergraduate degree in Psychology from the University of Dayton, and a Masters degree (religion, culture and business ethics) from Harvard University. Probably most importantly, she has spent months talking to people, including her Mom, about their perceptions of illness. They have shown through their words, laughter and tears that they identify deeply with what they've read in this book.

Living with PD may be Annie's burden, but writing about it is her passion!

NOTES

Printed in the United Kingdom
by Lightning Source UK Ltd.
121005UK00001B/70

9 781425 105181